WENDY MARQUENIE

Big Girl's PANTS

The Journey to Achieving Your Goal

Published by
Hasmark Publishing, judy@hasmarkservices.com

Disclaimer

This book is designed to provide information and motivation to our readers. It is sold with the understanding that the publisher is not engaged to render any type of psychological, legal, or any other kind of professional advice. The content of each article is the sole expression and opinion of its author, and not necessarily that of the publisher. No warranties or guarantees are expressed or implied by the publisher's choice to include any of the content in this volume. Neither the publisher nor the individual author(s) shall be liable for any physical, psychological, emotional, financial, or commercial damages, including, but "not limited to, special, incidental, consequential or other damages. Our views and rights are the same: You are responsible for your own choices, actions, and results.

Permission should be addressed in writing to Wendy Marquenie at marqueniew@gmail.com

Editor:
Sigrid Macdonald
Book Magic
http://bookmagic.biz

Cover and Book Design:
Anne Karklins
annekarklins@gmail.com

First Edition, 2018

ISBN-13: 978-1-988071-94-7
ISBN-10: 1988071941

Hasmark
PUBLISHING

I DEDICATE THIS BOOK to Bob Proctor and Sandy Gallagher and the Programs they have developed to educate and inspire each and every one of us to draw from within that which is truly inspirational. My book is the realization of an idea and a goal.

To all those who have yet to realize their dreams – let's travel on this journey together to fulfill lifelong desires and goals. To be the best you can be for yourself. To be the you that you want to be not the you that others would have you be.

Acknowledgements

SPECIAL THANKS TO Bob Proctor and Sandy Gallagher and the Proctor Gallagher Institute. Bob and Sandy are truly inspirational and great mentors in the area of personal development and growth.

SPECIAL THANKS TO my coach and mentor, Mario Piccone, for his excellent coaching and guidance.

SPECIAL THANKS TO my publisher, Judy O'Beirn and the team from Hasmark Services, for their guidance, advice, and their excellent service.

When you are surrounded by people with such knowledge and expertise in their respective areas, wonderful things begin to happen.

My Story

I CHOSE THE TITLE *Big Girl's Pants* because I thought it was appropriate for the information that I wanted to share and, having been there, I completely understand the frustrations associated with unattained desires and goals.

Sometimes circumstances and life require you to pull something out of you that you did not know was there. They require you to focus and get on with the job at hand. To be inspired and not doubt your abilities – this requires … Big Girl's Pants!

I wanted to share my journey from conference to achieving my goal.

Table of Contents

Acknowledgements iv

My Story v

Foreword 7

Chapter 1 9
Home from that Conference

Chapter 2 13
Developing Good Habits/Paradigms

Chapter 3 19
Goal Setting
How to Set a Goal

Chapter 4 23
Understanding The Laws of The Universe

Chapter 5 25
Universal Laws

Chapter 6 29
Intellectual Faculties of the Mind
Reason, Perception, Imagination, Will, Intuition, Memory

Chapter 7 33
Living in Harmony with The Laws

Chapter 8 37
Attitude

Chapter 9 39
Gratitude

Chapter 10 41
Self-Image

Chapter 11 45
Persistence & Study

Chapter 12 49
Conclusion

Chapter 13 53
In Summary

References 54
About the Author 55

Foreword

By Mario Piccone

AS I HAVE encountered and worked with many people over the past nine years in the personal development space, there is a very common thread among 97% of the world's population.

That is, as my mentor Bob Proctor says, "Many people tip toe their way through life, hoping they make it safely to their death."

But Wendy decided she would not be part of the 97% and instead be a part of the 3% club that actually make a decision and take action!

That's when I had the honor to meet Wendy at a live event in Toronto, Ontario in December 2016 – The Matrixx. It was the starting point of a great friendship and an opportunity to mentor her and watch her grow.

The book you are about to read is about a person who made a decision during a life changing live event and backed that up by taking action!

In this book, you will read and learn a number of very critical concepts that if applied consistently and persistently will literally change your life!

It has mine. It has Wendy's. AND if you decide and take action – It could for YOU TOO!

Begin your journey on the path to personal growth and...

Put on your "Big Girl's Pants"!

Enjoy!

With gratitude,

Mario
Piccone Coaching Inc.

Chapter 1

Home from that Conference

YOU HAVE RETURNED from that conference. You are excited as you have your goal set in your mind. The conference was absolutely fantastic. You met so many people and chatted about all the things you wanted to achieve. The adrenaline was in full speed, your heart was racing, and you knew this was a new beginning. This time you are going to make it. You can feel it. The conference was full on and many subjects were covered in its duration.

Maybe there were some follow-up exercises and reading you have to do. Maybe you have signed up for a couple of courses that require study and reading.

For the first few days, life is going well and you are very well organized and extremely committed to the tasks at hand. You keep thinking about the many things you learned at the conference. You are following the plan. Suddenly, on a particular day, you do not seem to fit into your schedule the work you were supposed to do. Then a few more days pass by and life seems to get far too busy. You tell yourself that you will catch up tomorrow, but tomorrow never comes. For some reason or another, you have more excuses. Why? You look around and that little voice in your head starts to mutter all kinds of questions. What are you doing? You can't do this. There is too much studying to do. You do not understand this program. You don't have the resources. You don't have the money. And so on and so on.

It is all well and good when you are with other like-minded people; the collaborative confidence inspired you and you became confident in your dream. You told yourself you could do it, but now that is a different story as you are back home.

You don't know where to start or you signed up for a particular program and it is not working out for you. That confidence dissipates and you let your dream die a very slow death along with your desire. You know you want to succeed, but that little voice in your head is taking over your thoughts and it is winning. That voice is playing a game in your Conscious Mind.

Those voices inside your head are significant. The only trouble is we invariably listen to the wrong voice messages.

Why do so many people not follow through with their dreams? They are so passionate about them in the beginning, but something stops them from making it happen. You might have been in this situation in the past. You know you do not want to follow the same path as before.

Believe me, I know. I have been here so many times in the past. I have attended many conferences that really got me excited and I couldn't wait to get home and get started, but that excitement soon faded. I found it difficult completing tasks especially when there was no one looking over my shoulder to guide me, mentor me and tell me that I have the ability to do it. I then started to put things off till the next day, then another day and another day and soon I lost interest. That desire I had in the beginning just faded away. I joined up with certain programs that were supposed to generate an income and when it did not generate any income, I again felt as if I had spent all this money and time learning something that did not work. I kept asking myself why it was not working.

For quite a few years I, unfortunately, followed this pattern and I thought I was a failure. I even had my family telling me that I had tried so many different things and none of them was successful and none of them earned an income. I felt really down because I did not know why I had not become that successful person or did not have a successful business and bring in the money that was supposed to happen. It seemed so easy for others to do it. Why didn't it happen for me?

I was given a book to read by Bob Proctor called *You Were Born Rich*. I diligently read every chapter and followed all the instructions. The more I read, the more excited I became. This was so unlike me as I have never been interested in reading books, but this time, something was different. I became hungry for more information and listened to many of Bob Proctor's YouTube videos. This information was so fascinating and I wanted to know more.

It wasn't until I studied a Proctor Gallagher Institute program called "Thinking Into Results" that I learned and understood why I lost interest in these different projects. I realized that many of the conferences that I had attended over the years concentrated only on the outside, instead of finding out the real reason why I was blocked from the inside (namely, my mind and the way I was thinking).

I now understand why I have not been the success I so desired and the reasons for writing this book so that I can share this information with you and help you understand why you do the things that you do and how you can change to achieve that success in your life.

There are plenty of seminars and conferences out there that might concentrate on creative concepts and information that will start you on the physical journey to success, but they do not emphasize the mental journey to success. One will not happen without the other. And until you understand the reasons why you have not succeeded in the past, life will forever remain the same.

Chapter 2

Developing Good Habits/Paradigms

TO FIRST SUCCEED IN LIFE, you have to understand yourself from the inside out. Your results are a reflection of your thoughts and your actions. By that I mean, take a look at what you are thinking about because you become what you think about all day long. If you have been thinking negative thoughts, you will have negative results. Your mind is a very powerful force and it is here that you need to change first before anything on the outside changes. Remember earlier when I spoke about those voices inside your head and how you are listening to the wrong messages? Up till now, you have been listening and following these voices and believing them. We live in a world through our senses; we have the ability to hear, see, smell, taste and touch. Throughout the day, many thoughts come flooding in through these senses and it is these thoughts that are controlling our way of thinking and acting. We have lived to react to these senses and have developed some particular habits/paradigms that have been detrimental to our success in life.

The secret to success is to understand how to integrate the knowledge that we have gathered during our lifetime with our behavioral patterns.

What are paradigms? Paradigms are a multitude of habits that we have formed since birth. Our whole life is habitual. When we first wake up in the morning, we do things without thinking about them. We follow the same pattern. We do not think about dressing or cleaning our teeth, do we? No, we just do them by habit.

When a baby is born, their Conscious Mind has not developed, but their Subconscious Mind is wide open. Environmentally through the five senses – hear, see, taste, touch, and smell – and genetically from our parents and grandparents, all of this contributes to the paradigms or habits that have developed. Why do you think we like and eat the same food as our parents? Why do we often think the same as our parents? This is where the image we have of ourselves is born, in the early stages of life through people, radio, television and family.

You can understand why these paradigms are such an important part of our life and our results in our life to this moment. If as a baby, we were subjected to a bad or negative upbringing, these paradigms are formed and we grow up behaving in a certain way.

Let us now dig further into our mind to discover why we think and act in a certain way. Because we think in pictures, we need a picture of our mind. Our mind is an activity, not a thing, and it is in every cell of our body. Let us, for a moment, think that our head is our mind, just for the purpose of this exercise, as we need a picture to work with as we think in pictures.

If we draw a large circle, draw a line across the middle and divide this circle into two, the top part of the circle will represent our Conscious Mind and bottom part of the circle represents our Subconscious Mind. Now the Conscious Mind is our thinking mind, our educated mind and it is the location for our intellect. The Conscious Mind has the ability to choose, accept or reject anything that flows into it. Over the years, we gather information from our school and higher learning, life experiences and through our sensory factors (hear, see, taste, touch and smell). Even though we have all this information and we know how to succeed, that doesn't mean that we are going to do it.

Our Subconscious Mind is the emotional mind. This is the part that controls our behavior and causes us to do what we do. In other words, it causes us to behave in a certain way. Whatever we plant in our Subconscious Mind grows. The Subconscious Mind must accept everything that is planted in it. It has no ability to choose. It cannot differentiate between what is real or imagined so any image we build, the Subconscious Mind will accept.

When we are talking about our paradigms or habits, these are fixed into our Subconscious Mind and here lies the answer to why we do and behave the way we do. This is the part of the mind that we need to focus on and change in order to achieve what we want in our life. Our Subconscious Mind operates by Law. It is the thoughts we think that produces the feelings we get and the actions we take to get the results we want. Remember when I said that whatever we think about, the Subconscious Mind holds onto that thought, so if I think about negative or bad results, that is the exact result I will get in life. That is operating by Law.

Andrew Carnegie once stated that: "Any idea that is held in the mind that was emphasized, either feared or revered will begin at once to clothe itself in the most convenient and appropriate physical form that was available."

In other words, any idea, whether it is a negative or positive, that you think about will produce those results in your life. Whatever you concentrate on comes into form. Take a look around you. What are the results you are currently getting in your life? Remember you become what you think about all day long.

How do we change these paradigms? The only way to change your paradigms that you have control over is through repetition. The other way that is forced upon you is by way of a sudden emotional impact and 99.99% of the time that is usually the result of bad news. So we won't focus on that here!

Write down a result that you are currently getting that you do not like. Change that result from a negative into a positive. Write the new paradigm down every day and read it every day because it is this repetition that fixes the new idea into your Subconscious Mind.

Continual space repetition, reading the same thing, writing the same thing and listening to the same thing over and over. This positive repetition becomes fixed in our Subconscious Mind and gradually becomes stronger than the negative one and the positive result takes over. That is the only way for you to change your results.

Persist with this activity until you achieve the desired result. Persistence – the ability to give yourself a command and follow it. The lack of persistence is one of the major causes of failure. If you find that you have difficulty keeping yourself to task, seek out someone who will be your accountability buddy; that way they will keep you focused and on track.

"Paradigms are powerful because they create the
lens through which we see the world."
– Napoleon Hill

Conclusion and Notes:

1. Write down a paradigm that you wish to change and replace it with a positive one.

_____

_____

_____

_____

_____

_____

_____

_____

2. Be persistent. Write it down every day and read it every day.

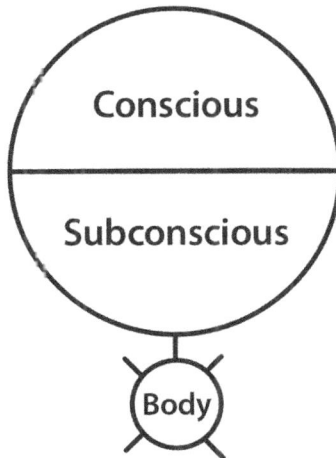

Chapter 3

Goal Setting
How to Set a Goal

I THINK THE BEST DEFINITION of a goal was by Earl Nightingale when he stated that: "Success is the progressive realization of a worthy goal."

Studying this material enabled me to finally understand the reasons why I had not achieved anything I tried in the past. I was going after the wrong goal. I thought it was my dream and the right goal. Looking back and thinking about it, I can say now that it really wasn't something that I truly wanted to do in my life. I thought it was at the time. I did not have that burning desire in my belly to succeed. I only thought I wanted it.

How do we set a goal? A goal is something that you are going after that you have never done before. Remember when setting a goal, it has to be a great big goal: a goal that you do not know how you will get there. One that you really, really, really want. One that turns you on so much and that the desire to get there is so overwhelming, nothing will stop you from achieving it.

Your ultimate goal is to grow from within, have faith and believe that you are ready to accept it.

For me, it is a fire in my belly. I get so excited and happy and cannot wait to start every new day to see how close I can get to achieving my goal. This excitement takes over my whole body. This is the feeling I am talking about.

When people say that they do not know what they want, I do not believe that is a true statement.

They say that because they have not sat down and truly thought about it. You have an abundance of creativity within you and now is the time to draw on that power.

Find a quiet place, let your mind wander, fantasize, start to imagine and build that picture in your mind of what you want. See yourself in that fantasy. Look around you. This is like a movie about your life and you are creating this movie just how you want it to be. This is the picture you are going to impress upon your Subconscious Mind because, as we established before, your Subconscious Mind has no ability to reject and it cannot tell whether something is real or imagined.

You are excited about your life's movie. Your body is reacting to this excitement and the feelings you are experiencing because your body is an instrument of the mind. You are at this minute becoming emotionally involved with this idea. This sets off a chain reaction. This is how the Law works. The minute you become emotionally involved in the idea, your idea now becomes a goal and The Universe conspires to start the flow of events to make this happen.

When I was contemplating what to do for the rest of my life, I started to think about what I loved to do more than anything else. I came up with two things, dancing and traveling, so I had to figure out how to incorporate these two together to find something that really turned me on. I must admit it did take a few weeks to figure it out. I came up with a number of ideas and the more I thought about it, I realized that some of these ideas would not work so I got rid of those. Then one day I came up with an idea of how to incorporate them together. My business and website name was born: www.shapeupforsuccess.com – having a Healthy Mind and Body, developing a Healthy Mind through The Proctor Gallagher Institute programs and a Healthy Body through the proper use of the mind and my movement through music videos. I fantasized about taking this concept to the world. I was so happy and excited. This generated a fire within me; I became emotionally involved in this idea. I took action immediately. I finally found my journey just as you can.

If your goal is not turning out the way you expect, then you have to rethink it. Ask yourself what is it that you truly love to do, e.g., traveling, walking, going to the gym, becoming a teacher, helping people? How can you take what you love to do and do it every single day for the rest of your life? Write it down and then start to dream of it in pictures as if it is here already and you are living your dream. How does that make you feel? Very excited, I bet. As you become emotionally involved in your idea, this is now becoming your goal. Are you able to turn your fantasy into your goal? Are you willing to do whatever it takes to reach your goal? Unless you take action and actually do something about it, your goal will remain only as a fantasy.

When you don't have a goal, the outside world is controlling you. You are lost. When you do have a goal, you are controlling the outside world. You have a purpose.

Conclusion and Notes:

We have to have a goal to keep us moving forward. Without a goal, we are lost; we have no direction in our life.

1. Write down your goal (the date of your goal might change, but your goal remains the same).

My goal is

_____

_____

Date _____

I am so happy and grateful now that…

_____

_____

_____

_____

_____

2. Read it every day to plant the picture in your Subconscious Mind.

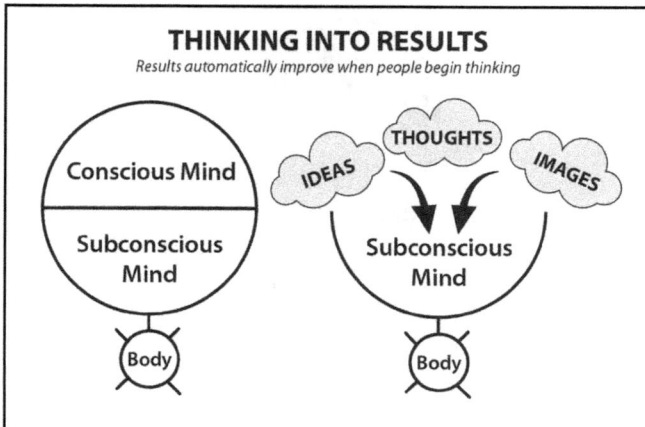

THINKING INTO RESULTS
Results automatically improve when people begin thinking

Conscious Mind

Subconscious Mind

Body

IDEAS   THOUGHTS   IMAGES

Subconscious Mind

Body

Chapter 4

Understanding The Laws of The Universe

EVERYTHING IS OUT THERE in The Universe and all of the inventions over time have always been out there just waiting for someone to grab their idea and make it happen. You can make your dream or idea materialize. You are the only person that can do that. You have an abundance of creativity within you and now is the time to draw on that power.

Understand that the very moment you decide to move forward with your idea, you start a chain reaction. You become excited, your energy levels increase, you begin to change the way you think, you become positive that it will work out, you have that excited feeling running through your body and that vibration is sent out into The Universe. The Universe reacts to this and just like magic, it all starts to happen. Remember how you were feeling at the conference? You were pumped about your idea, you were positive, you were excited, you couldn't wait to get home and get started.

Wouldn't you like to have that same feeling permanently? You can. You can have anything you set your mind to.

I mentioned briefly earlier about The Universe. The Universe is governed by Laws and we must follow these Laws to receive what we desire.

I know what you are thinking. Do not tune out on me now. When I first heard about these Laws, I too rolled my eyes and thought to myself, what a load of codswallop. I was naive because I did not understand. So I decided to research and do a little bit of study because this is important information that I needed to know. I wanted to know how The Laws work and how I can use them effectively to achieve my desires in life.

If we do not understand and follow these Laws exactly, we can work at something and put everything we have into it, but success will elude us. To be rich, we have to do things in a certain way. There is a science to getting rich. The Laws of The Universe are exact. The Laws work exactly the same way every time for every single person. If that is the case, then each of us has the ability to achieve what we want just like all the people that we consider successful. They became successful by thinking and doing things in a certain way.

Let's take a look at these Laws and try to understand them.

Chapter 5
Universal Laws

THERE ARE CERTAIN LAWS of The Universe that we must understand and follow. If you want to achieve anything of significance, you must obey these Laws as they are exact. The Laws are connected to one another. These Laws are so precise that they work the same for every person every time. There is a science to getting rich which is how The Universe operates. There are 7 Universal Laws of Success:

1. Law of Perpetual Transmutation of Energy
2. Law of Vibration and Attraction
3. Law of Relativity
4. Law of Polarity
5. Law of Rhythm
6. Law of Cause and Effect
7. Law of Gender

Law of Perpetual Transmutation of Energy

If we take a look at the Law of Perpetual Transmutation of Energy – what does that mean? We know energy is movement and everything is constantly moving. Energy is in every cell of our body. Energy is continually moving into form and through form and back into form. If we study energy looking at a year cycle of a bush, in spring the leaves come out, the buds and flowers come out. Then in autumn, the leaves fall off and the buds and flowers fall off. Nature is continually moving in a cycle of energy. The energy in the tree is continually moving in harmony with The Laws of Nature.

Every thought we think about during the day is always moving in and out of our Conscious Mind. When we think, we build images, and these images move into form into our Conscious Mind. Whatever you concentrate on immediately starts to move into form.

The Law of Vibration and Attraction

This is a very powerful Law as this is where like attracts like. The Law of Vibration is the primary Law and the Law of Attraction is the secondary Law. This Law is always working.

The Law of Attraction states that:

"The **law of attraction** is the attractive, magnetic power of the Universe that draws similar energies together. It manifests through the power of creation, everywhere and in many ways. Even the **law** of gravity is part of the **law of attraction**. This **law** attracts thoughts, ideas, people, situations and circumstances." (Definition provided by Remez Sasson on the website Success Consciousness, in the article "The Law of Attraction – Meaning and Definition.")

1. ASK for what you want and The Universe will manifest what you are feeling by rearranging itself to make it happen.

2. BELIEVE (with complete sincerity) that you already have what you want and The Universe will answer.

3. RECEIVE it and be grateful that your request was granted. You must bring yourself into alignment in order to receive. Find the feeling and it will manifest itself into form to and through you.

Think, Feel, Manifest – The Universe is like a genie: "Your Wish Is My Command." The moment you begin to think properly, The Universe will guide you if you let it. Everything is energy and by changing the energy, The Universe will change also.

How do you feel today? Our body is moving on a certain vibration. Some days we might be feeling a little low and then other days, we have endless amounts of energy. We have the ability to alter the vibration we are in. So when you are not feeling great one day, you can change and alter that vibration. Play some music that will get you up and dancing around. Do whatever it takes to alter that state you are in.

The Law of Relativity

This is the Law of Comparison. It is how one thing is compared to other things. Hot exits because we compare it to cold. Good exists because we compare that to bad. Everything is the same until we compare it to something else. Everything just is until it is compared to something else. There is no big or small, fast or slow except by comparison.

Take a look at your results, or what you are doing, and compare this to what you are capable of doing. Think about how you can improve your actions that will lead you to your goal.

The Laws of Polarity

Everything in The Universe has an opposite and cannot function otherwise. Hot and cold, up and down, good and bad, positive and negative. When we fail at something, that generally means we will then succeed at something.

We should always be looking for the good in every situation we encounter and also the people we come in contact with. Imagine how that person would feel if you complimented them on a particular thing. That would instantly make them feel good and, consequently, more positive. Good compliment equals an increase in good vibration.

The Law of Rhythm

Everything in The Universe is moving just like a dance, to and fro, backward and forward. There is always a reaction to every action that you take. The world we live in moves within the Law of Rhythm; night follows day and tides come in and go out. We also live in a state of rhythm intellectually, emotionally and physically. If you are experiencing something bad, you know and understand that there is a better one to follow. Give more to each day so that each day will be the best you can give for that day.

The Law of Cause and Effect

What is coming into your life is a reflection of yourself. This Law is considered the Law of all Laws. Everything that happens to us happens according to Law. Whatever you are sending out into The Universe comes back. Action and reaction. There is a saying, "What you sow, you will reap." This is your attitude. It is how you treat others and how others will treat you. If you treat everyone you come in contact with well, it will come back to you. Only concentrate on what you can give to others rather than what you can get from them.

The Law of Gender

This is the creative Law. The Laws states that "Everything in nature is both male and female and both are required for life to exist." Nothing in The Universe is created or destroyed. Everything is already here waiting for someone to pluck it out. The way to build a plane or create computers has always been here. It just needed for someone to manifest it. Everything is created twice, once in the mind and once in the physical sense. Everything has a gestation or incubation period, just like a baby takes nine months from conception to birth, or seeds to grow into a flower or tree. The same applies to everything we want in our life. It will have a gestation period before it arrives. Do not give up on your goal too early. Let the amount of time pass before it manifests for you. By concentrating on your goal, this increases energy and in turn shortens the gestation span.

All Laws relate to each other. Everything operates in an orderly fashion by Law. Everything is possible when you know how to apply The Laws of The Universe. This is where our intellectual faculties come into play. Focus your attention on the objective you want to reach.

Chapter 6

Intellectual Faculties of the Mind
Reason, Perception, Imagination, Will, Intuition, Memory

LET'S LOOK AT these wonderful mental tools and learn to develop them. Start to observe what is going on around you.

Reason – this is our ability to think and choose. We can be taught how to think just the same way we can be taught to learn a language or play an instrument. Thinking taps into the infinite. We create thoughts which are pictures; we join them all together and that is how we build an idea. An idea is just a collection of thoughts directed toward a purpose. You must not let what is going on in the outside control your mind.

Dr. Ryan stated that: "The mind is the greatest power in all of creation." Look at the results you are getting right now and if you do not like these results, think about how you can do better. Think about what you want and build that image to make it a reality. Thoughts and ideas cause the feeling, which causes the actions which produces the new results. We can either react or respond. When you react to things going on outside, then they are in control of you, but when you respond to what is going on around you, then you maintain control. Look at your results, adapt and start with a new train of results, and that way you stay in charge of you.

Perception – perception is just a point of view. There are many ways of looking at everything in the world. If we see something and think why it cannot be done, let's change our point of view and work out how it can be done. Change your perception; then you will change your point of view.

Imagination – Napoleon Hill said: "Imagination is the most marvelous, miraculous, inconceivably powerful force the world has ever known."

Everything is built on imagination. Everything in this Universe is created twice, once in the imagination of your mind and then again in the outside world. Use your imagination to see how you can do things better. We use our imagination to look beyond where we are at.

Will – this is a fabulous tool to develop. With the power of your will, you are able to hold one picture on the screen of your mind to the exclusion of all outside distractions. The will makes your mind stronger. You use your will to stop all the things coming into our mind from the outside world through the sensory factors. The more you practice developing your will, the stronger it will become.

Intuition – we use our intuitive factor to pick up different vibrations from people. It helps you to feel and know what is happening around you. Sometimes when you meet a person for the first time and you get a funny feeling, you are picking up on the energy from this person. That is our intuitive factor. This mental muscle is like God is talking to us. We have to learn to get tuned in and use it as this will make us a more powerful, creative person and then we will obtain better results.

Memory – we have a fantastic memory. There is no such thing as a bad memory, only a weak memory. Are you like me? When I am introduced to someone and I have never seen them before, I always have trouble remembering their name. We can learn to improve our memory using the association method. To practice this method, when I am first introduced to someone, I try and think of something that would remind me of this person's name, e.g., If I were introduced to a person with the name of Doris, then I would associate this person with actress Doris Day. See what I mean? Try it for yourself. How we remember names is different from how we remember numbers.

Proper use of the intellectual factors is how we apply this Law of Attraction.

Learn to develop your mental faculties and observe what is going on around you. Develop your mental faculties to get what you want.

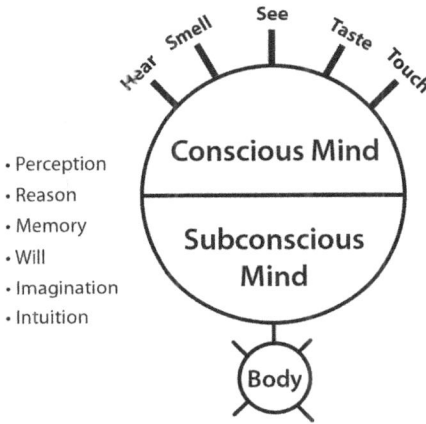

- Perception
- Reason
- Memory
- Will
- Imagination
- Intuition

Hear Smell See Taste Touch

Conscious Mind

Subconscious Mind

Body

BOLD BEAUTIFUL BLISSFUL U

Illustration originally designed by Dr. Thurman Fleet

Chapter 7

Living in Harmony with The Laws

WE HAVE TO LIVE IN HARMONY with The Laws for us to succeed and fulfill our dreams. To be in harmony with the Law of The Universe, we have to do things in a certain way.

We attract to us what we think about. If you have negative thoughts, then negativity is what you are attracting. Believe me, this is true. Have you ever been faced with a situation where you were thinking negatively and what you were worried about actually happened? You attracted the negative. Have you ever experienced waking up and not feeling all that great and then the whole day is disastrous? One thing after another goes wrong and you tell yourself you should have stayed home. Just think of how you could have changed the outcome of that day by changing your attitude from the moment you wake up. You can change your way of thinking from negative to positive by doing something that changes your mood. Do something you like, for example, playing some music that you really enjoy listening to. For me, I love to dance around the lounge room like no one is watching. That immediately shifts my thought pattern. Find something that works for you.

The movie *The Secret* talks about the Law of Attraction and how we think and how what we think about happens, whether we are thinking negative or positive thoughts. The secret is to replace negative with positive thoughts so that we get the results we want in life. I am not talking about all your thoughts. We have thoughts flowing through us all day long through our five sensory factors, which are hear, see, taste, touch and smell. We are bombarded with thoughts every day and a lot of them we do not register at all. They just come in and go out without notice. It is the important negative thoughts that we are entertaining that are controlling our emotions, our attitude, our self-image, our results with work, our relationships in life that we have to start to recognize and change. Look around you for a moment. The life you are leading right now you have created because we attract into our life what we think about. To change the results, we have to change the way we think.

The Law of Vibration and Attraction is one of the most powerful Laws and it is the one that we should really pay attention to and understand because unless we develop an understanding of how it works, we will never achieve our goals in life.

Think about your goal, what you desire the outcome to be. Start to imagine and visualize your life as if you have already achieved your goal. This sets up a different vibration that you are sending out into The Universe. Remember you do not have to know how you are going to get there; you just have to believe that you can. Things will present themselves as, and when, required. That is the Law. When you take action to move toward your goal, your goal will move toward you.

We are a mass of energy that is always moving. The whole Universe vibrates; nothing rests. Our body is continually moving on a particular frequency or vibration. Our body is vibrating on a certain frequency. Everything is connected; that is how you attract things into your life.

Think of our energy as lines horizontally drawn on a piece of paper at equal distances apart. Every frequency or vibration on that page is connected to the one above and the one below. We attract to us what is on the same frequency as ourselves. So if you want to attract something that is on a different higher frequency, then you have to increase your frequency or vibration to reach it. We have the ability to hook up with any frequency and by doing that, we can attract what we want into our life.

All creatures and plant life on this earth are programmed to grow in a certain way and don't have the ability to change how they grow. We are the only ones that can change our lives. All creatures on this earth are born to operate by instinct and are very comfortable with their surroundings. We are the only ones on this planet that are uncomfortable with our environment. All creatures already know what to do to survive. They know how to hunt and gather food for themselves. We, as babies, have to be taught how to do everything. All the animals live by the use of their sensory factors. The only way we differ from all these animals is by the use of our intellectual faculties of the mind – reason, perception, imagination, will, intuition and memory.

Proper use of the intellectual faculties is how we apply this Law of Attraction. We have been programmed through our upbringing to listen to what is going on in the outside world through our five sensory factors. The trouble is, we will never ever achieve anything of significance living this way, from the outside in. Learn to develop these mental faculties to serve you. Start to observe what is going on around you.

Chapter 8

Attitude

EARL NIGHTINGALE ONCE SAID that attitude was "The Magic Word."

Attitude is the foundation for success. Attitude is our thoughts, feelings and actions, which are expressed through the mind and body. The attitude we have toward others determines life's attitude toward us. Attitude determines the results you will get in life: the Law of Cause and Effect. Everything in life is controlled by Law.

We, as human beings, can alter our lives by altering our attitudes of mind, but the problem today is that people do not know how to do that.

Our attitude is a mind body thing and we need an image of the mind to work with to try and understand that by altering the mind, we can alter the vibration our body is in to put us on the same vibratory level as our goal.

Thoughts + Feelings + Actions = Results

Our feelings trigger actions, which produces results.

Our attitude is a reflection of what is going on – on the inside. Present results are the physical action of our past results. Do not let the present results control your future results.

If we go back to the drawing of the mind that I mentioned earlier, the large circle represents the mind, which is divided by a line. The upper is the

Conscious Mind and the bottom half is the Subconscious Mind. Because our Conscious Mind is the thinking mind, the educated mind and where our intellect is, it has the ability to accept, reject or ignore any thoughts or ideas and information that comes in through our sensory factors. What thoughts we have are entering our Conscious Mind. That determines what we place into our Subconscious Mind and flows into our body either through a negative or positive vibration.

Our Subconscious Mind is our emotional mind and can only accept what has been planted in there. It cannot differentiate between what is real and what is imagined. What is impressed into our Subconscious Mind controls the vibration of the body. The body is an instrument of the mind and will do exactly what the mind tells it to do. We need to control what is being planted into our Subconscious Mind.

If we break it down further, we gather thoughts that when combined form an idea which comes into our Conscious Mind. We turn that idea into a picture and plant it in our Subconscious Mind, recalling that our Subconscious Mind will accept anything we think about. When we become emotionally involved with this idea, it sets off a vibration in our body. This vibration will then dictate what is attracted back to us.

When you have a positive idea and internalize it, you move into a positive vibration and you will attract like energy to you. This is where you control you.

Positive thinkers get positive results.

Attitude is everything and attitude really is The Magic Word for creating success in life.

Chapter 9

Gratitude

HAVING AN ATTITUDE of gratitude changes everything.

When someone mentions to you about being grateful, we know we should be grateful for our life at present, but most times we are unsure why and what it really does for us.

Being grateful instantly shifts your way of thinking and your energy. It puts you in harmony with The Universe so that everything we desire in life moves toward us. Action – reaction.

Next time when everything doesn't seem to be going your way, just stop what you are doing and think about all the things in your life that you are grateful for. I know this might be a hard thing to do especially when your problems are dominating your every thought, but when you start feeling grateful for everything, life seems to shift immediately. When you change the way you are looking at the problems you are facing, then the problems will change.

Earl Nightingale in the series "Lead the Field" suggested that every morning we write down at least 10 things that we are grateful for.

I write what I am grateful for in my gratitude diary every day. This helps me to genuinely think about my life and what I have and what I have achieved. This exercise also puts me in a good vibration for the day. The Law of Cause and Effect – what you put out there comes back to you.

Gratitude: What are you grateful for?

I am so happy and grateful now that

_____

_____

_____

_____

_____

_____

_____

_____

Chapter 10
Self-Image

DR. MAXWELL MALTZ SAID that "Self-image sets the individual boundaries of our accomplishments."

The image we have of ourselves was created as a baby through our Subconscious Mind. All the information from the outside world from radio, television, other people and, of course, our relatives formed the picture of who we are way back then. These are our paradigms.

We go through life unaware of the image we have of ourselves, but we do not realize that this self-image influences every part of our life. If we have a negative image of ourselves, then our results in life will be negative. You can have a person who is well educated and extremely intelligent but has a very poor image of themselves.

We have a control mechanism in our mind and this determines what comes into our life and how well we do things. We, in fact, have two images: one that we project to the world by the way we talk, walk, dress, etc. and the other one is the picture we hold inside. The picture we hold on the inside definitely shows on the outside. Our results are always a reflection of what is going on inside.

Your life today is the result of your self-image that was created in your Subconscious Mind when you were a baby.

A confident individual has an understanding of who they are. They understand their personality, spiritually. They understand the power of their mind. They understand themselves and they like them themselves and have a good opinion and a good self-image.

Quite often our self-image is bogged down by paradigms, doubts about ourselves and insecurity. So how do we change our self-image? What image are you portraying to the outside world? To change our self-image, we again have to take a look at what paradigms we have locked up in our Subconscious Mind that are causing our self-image and change them.

Our life operates by images. This is where we put our mind to work. We consciously and deliberately choose the kind of person we want to be. Pick a quality or character trait of a person we really admire and envision yourself being that person. Sit down and write a description in the present tense of your self-image. Internalize it and see yourself as that person as if you are acting in your own movie. Be that person.

When I think about my self-image, I think about this picture of a small kitten looking into a mirror and the image it reflects back is one of a big lion. I think I resonate so much with that image because I am not very tall or large in stature. The biggest problem with the image I used to see in the mirror of myself was of the small kitten. Over the years, I have tried different ventures and none of them was successful in any way. I did not believe that I was smart enough. I thought that only people who had money and had come from a business like background were successful in life. I did not grow up being exposed to either of those things. I did not believe that I could ever achieve all the goals that I had set for myself at the conference.

Let me ask you this:

What is the reflection you see of yourself when you look in the mirror?

Do you like what you see?

Is it one of self-doubt in your own ability to succeed in anything you desire to achieve?

What is holding you back from going forward?

The past doesn't own you. You can get up and walk out at any time.

You know you are quite capable of changing the direction of your life and in order to do that, you have to belief in yourself.

Don't let your paradigms destroy your self-image. Empower and discipline your mind to a successful life.

Start creating this wonderful life you want. Learn to love yourself, be good to yourself. Get in touch with you. There is something wonderful about you.

See it – your self-image.

Write down a description of your self-image…

_____

_____

_____

_____

_____

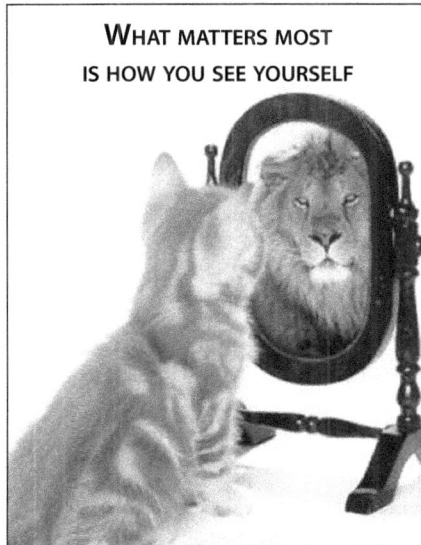

WHAT MATTERS MOST IS HOW YOU SEE YOURSELF

Chapter 11
Persistence & Study

IN THE BOOK by Napoleon Hill, *Think and Grow Rich*, he talks about persistence as a state of mind and therefore something that can be cultivated. To develop persistence, you need to have a definite purpose along with the desire that is so strong that nothing will stop you from fulfilling that goal.

Know what your goal is and take action to acquire it. Do not listen to anything negative. Remain positive and focused and have someone to encourage you to follow through with your goal.

Persistence is essential in order to achieve all that you desire to achieve in life. It is this lack of persistence that is one of the main causes of failure.

Persistence requires the use of one of our intellectual factors, which is the will. Will power and desire, when combined, are unstoppable in achieving goals.

Napoleon Hill states that the starting point of all achievement is DESIRE. Weak desires bring weak results.

Remember back when we were setting a goal.

Our goal is something that we want so badly that there is inside us that desire to achieve it. Desire is that fire in your belly that urges you to take action so that this big goal will be achieved. If that desire is not there, all your efforts will be in vain. It just will not happen.

If you have created that picture of your goal in your mind, you now use your will to keep that picture firmly planted there. That will also ignite the fire because you are getting excited about it. Can you see by having that picture firmly planted in your Subconscious Mind that your body has increased its vibration level to seek out the same level as your goal? Your mind and body are now moving closer toward it. Use your persistence habit to keep that fire burning. Persistence has to be developed; it is not something that comes naturally. If you find that you are wavering in persistence, find a friend or a group of friends to keep you on track when you start to wobble. When you develop a good habit of persistence, nothing will stop you from succeeding and achieving.

Here are some simple steps to develop a consistent habit of persistence:

1. Make sure your goal is something that you are emotionally connected to, something that you really desire to achieve.

2. Take action immediately toward your goal. As your goal becomes more defined, a pathway to accomplishing it will become more apparent.

3. Do not allow any negative thoughts from the outside world to stop you deviating from your path toward your goal.

4. Have a friend or group of friends around you that will offer support if and when needed to keep you on that journey to success.

Persistence is a wonderful mental strength to acquire because it is this strength that we will draw on when at first we do not succeed. Persistence is the one thing that we need to call upon to keep going until our goal is achieved. We must prepare ourselves for the possibility that the outcome may not be what we desire the first time around. Life happens and we sometimes are faced with uncertainty and obstacles.

If we look back in history, people like Sir Edmund Hillary tried to climb Mount Everest three times; on the last attempt, he was successful. He conquered the mountain and reached the top. Thomas Edison repeatedly worked on the incandescent light bulb 10,000 times before he was successful. When asked why he kept going, he said, "I have not failed. I've just found 10,000 ways that won't work." – Thomas A. Edison

So take heed and learn a lesson from this. Do not give up at the first sign of difficulties. Keep that desire burning and you will succeed.

Persistence, concentration of effort and definiteness of purpose are the major sources of all achievements.

Study – you might be wondering, why is study important to achieve anything in this life?

In order to achieve anything, we first must study. If we choose to go to university or college or to attain an apprenticeship, we must study that particular course in order to pass. If we wish to be the best in our field, we need to study so that we become a master of our chosen career.

We can have all the knowledge stacked up like books in our Conscious Mind and still not achieve anything in life. Why? I am endeavoring through these chapters to educate you on the powers of the mind and how our mind controls everything in our life. It is at this point in our life, we have become what we think about. I can be the most intelligent person in the world, but if I do not understand how my mind operates in connection to my outside world, then I will achieve nothing of significance. I study to become the master of my mind and how it works.

How am I supposed to change my habits/paradigms that I have developed since my infant days without study? It is the continuous reading, writing and listening to the same things every day that plant good, successful habits into my Subconscious Mind that will help me attain my goals. I study to learn how to get rid of all negative thoughts and replace them with positive because I know that is what I need to do to reach my goal. It is the repetitive learning that seeps into the Subconscious Mind and changes my world. Remember the Subconscious Mind has no ability to reject – it will accept anything and everything I put in there. The reason why we go over the same things is because we do not necessarily have 100% focus when we are reading, writing or listening the first time around. Our mind drifts in and out. I know I have listened to a particular recording many times and there will be one occasion when I will hear something that I swear I have never heard before. When we were discussing paradigms/habits and how to change them, we wrote out the positive and then read them every day for a while. The same with your goal card.

Make study a success habit every single day.

Chapter 12

Conclusion

I KNOW WHEN I ARRIVED back home from my conference, there was so much to think about, so much to do. I had two projects that I was working on at the same time. I made contact with the people who offered to help me with my projects. I have two medium sized white boards: one for each project. I wrote down a list of everything that had to be completed and as I went through them and completed each one, I place a big tick next to it. By doing this, I stayed focused on the tasks at hand. Yes, I did have some setbacks along the way, but when that happened, I refocused on the problem. When I did that, I discovered an alternate path to take and then continued again to complete the goal I had set for myself.

If you experience little setbacks, don't let indecision, doubt and fear take over. Napoleon Hill in his book, *Think and Grow Rich*, stated that INDECISION is the seedling of FEAR. Indecision crystalizes into DOUBT. The two blend together to turn into FEAR. This fear comes from our Subconscious Mind, which causes us to become anxious throughout the body. When you are indecisive, you start to doubt yourself and your ability to go through with your goal. This feeling then creates the fear and anxiety. Why the three of these are so dangerous is because they creep up on you slowly without you knowing it. You must work through this. These fears are just states of mind. Faith is the opposite of fear. We all have these thoughts that come into our lives, especially when we are working on our goal and this is where you must have faith in your ability, faith in yourself.

So why is this time any different? I asked myself. This time I knew where I was going wrong and how to change it. I had to change the way I was thinking. I completed the "Thinking Into Results" program and put into practice all that I had learned. I continued to study every day because it is the repetition that causes you to believe.

I learned about the paradigms I had of myself that were stopping me from achieving my goals. I learned how to change the way I was thinking and my behavior. It is an ongoing process, one that I will work on now every single day of my life. I know I have to maintain the study to keep learning and to continually remember the power of my mind. When life is not going according to plan, I now know that if I re-evaluate the situation, I will find a better way. I re-evaluate my thoughts and actions.

My journey hasn't always gone according to plan. I have recently had a major disappointment and setback and I must admit, it did throw me for a six. I did struggle for quite a few days and questioned a lot of information that I had been studying. The Law of Attraction states that it works the same for every person every single time. Well, on this occasion, the Law of Attraction did not work and I questioned why. I built the picture, I planted it in my Subconscious Mind, I internalized it. I became so emotionally involved and thought about it every day and when it did not turn out the way I desired – I was so distraught. I had to sit down and really analyze the situation. I had to dig deep. I pondered and thought and walked (whenever I have a problem or situation, when I go for a walk, it seems to clear my head and open up my thoughts).

Earl Nightingale in his "Lead the Field" recordings stated that when this type of situation happens, we might not know the reasons why, but we must have faith that something better is just around the corner. It is not always easy to hold your faith and have belief that all will turn out in the end, but that is exactly what you have to do. That is exactly what I had to do. I do have faith in my ability to achieve my goal and I certainly will not quit at this point. I will continue on my path to achievement. My journey is continuing; that is for sure.

There is a famous quote by Vincent Lombardi – "Winners never quit and quitters never win."

Life is a very interesting journey when you know how to navigate properly through the recesses of your mind. I never knew that success could be obtained so easily, just by learning how The Mind and The Universe works.

Create the life you want. Be the best that you can be.

Pull up those Big Girl's Pants and get the job done.

DREAM   CREATE   BUILD   ENJOY

"Learn to enjoy every minute of your life.
Be happy now. Don't wait for something outside of yourself to
make you happy in the future. Think how really precious is
the time you have to spend, whether it's at work or with your family.
Every minute should be enjoyed and savored."
– Earl Nightingale

Chapter 13

In Summary

1. Change your paradigms one at a time.

2. Think about your goal and write it out on a card – a goal that is so big it excites and scares you at the same time. Read your goal every day. EMOTIONALIZE YOURSELF WITH IT.

3. Start developing the faculties of your mind – Reason, Perception, Imagination, Will, Intuition AND Memory.

4. Attitude – having an excellent attitude will produce excellent results.

5. Write in your gratitude diary every day, all that you are grateful for.

6. Now that you have written down a description of your self-image – read it every day and become that person – this is your movie!

7. Be persistent – write a list of actions and study and do this every day.

8. Find a mentor who will guide you to success.

References

THANK YOU TO Bob Proctor and Sandy Gallagher and the programs that they have developed to educate and encourage each and every one of us to draw from within that which is truly inspirational.

Reference material from The Proctor Gallagher Institute programs:
- Thinking Into Results
- The New Lead The Field
- The Matrixx Conference

And the following books:
Think and Grow Rich by Napoleon Hill
The Science of Getting Rich by Wallace D. Wattles
Working With The Law by Raymond Holliwell
You Were Born Rich by Bob Proctor

Contact details:
Wendy Marquenie
Website: www.shapeupforsuccess.com
Email: marqueniew@gmail.com

Please contact me if you have an interest in learning more about any of the above programs. I would be happy to be of service and mentor you on your road to success.

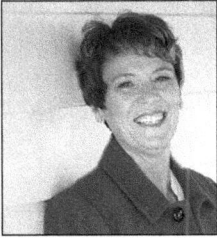

About the Author

I HAVE ALWAYS HAD AN INTEREST in dancing, and at an early age, I commenced classes in tap and ballet. Through these years, I gained many accolades and even a scholarship and always found dancing to be lots of fun and quite easy.

Marriage, divorce, motherhood and raising a family bring along its own set of challenges, and the years quickly flew by. I commenced studies in a different form of dance, Latin/Ballroom, and became a qualified professional teacher and adjudicator. During the many years that followed, I enjoyed many additional careers choices, as a travel consultant and in airline customer service and flight attendant roles.

A major life challenge presented itself, and as I worked through the many issues, I found myself looking for my next career move. I was sent a free book, You Were Born Rich by Bob Proctor. I was so fascinated by the material in the book that I wanted to learn more. I signed up for the Thinking Into Results Program, had a wonderful coach, Mario Piccone, and attended The Matrixx in Toronto, December 2016. I wrote this book to share my experiences with the world. My website: www.shapeupforsuccess. com is being developed. I enjoy helping people to develop healthy minds through the Proctor Gallagher programs as well as developing healthy bodies through my dance exercise videos and nutritional information.

My journey is just beginning.

Wendy Marquenie has just released
How to Change Your Life in Six Days.

"I had the pleasure to coach Wendy... there was such a dramatic change to her which clearly allowed her to take things to the next level while at The Matrixx. Wendy is very focused and driven to create the success she expects and deserves! Well done, Wendy."

~ Mario Piccone, Coaching & Training Coordinator,
Proctor Gallagher Institute

As a dance teacher, Wendy Marquenie came up with an idea of how she could best help others by combining her two passions; combine a healthy mind with a healthy body.

How and what we think will ultimately affect our results of achieving anything in life. She teaches we need to learn to love yourself; be good to yourself because our mind controls everything in our life. You have to believe in yourself and your ability to achieve as we all have the ability to nurture our dreams, goals and aspirations. Make a difference not only for yourself but for the next generation.

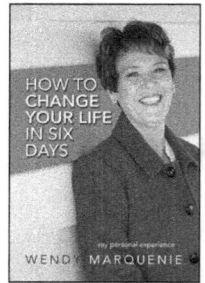

Transform your life; bring out the creative power you have within you. You are the most magnificent expressions of life.

"Open your mind and be ready to experience positive change in your life... When you do, your life will never be the same. I have always had an interest in dancing, and with Wendy's book combining the two, it allowed me to once again enjoy it. My journey is just beginning, through Wendy's book, let yours begin as well."

~ Peggy McColl, *New York Times* Best Selling Author

To learn more about the book or for information on receiving your own copy, please reach out to Wendy:

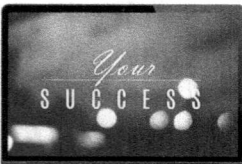

Email: **marqueniew@gmail.com**
Website: **www.shapeupforsuccess.com**

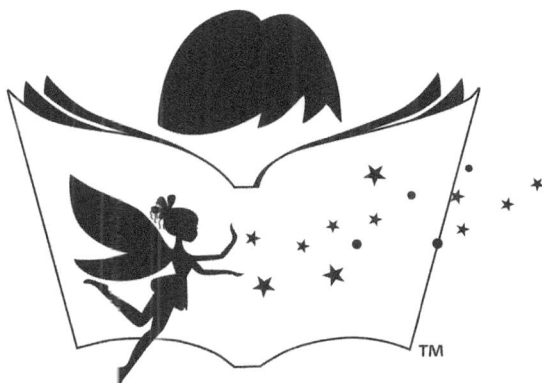

THE LITERARY FAIRIES

We make your literary wish come true!

Wendy Marquenie

has partnered with

The Literary Fairies

Their mission is to grant literary wishes to those who have experienced or are experiencing an adversity in their life or have a disability and wish to share their story with the world to uplift, inspire and entertain through literacy.

Visit TLF website to find out how YOU could have your literary wish granted or if you wish to make a donation.

More details provided at
www.theliteraryfairies.com

www.ingramcontent.com/pod-product-compliance
Lightning Source LLC
Chambersburg PA
CBHW072021290326
41934CB00009BA/2151